A Complete Guideline About

Binge Eating Disorder

By

Martin G

The goal of this book is to offer accurate and reliable information about the subject at hand. The publisher is not obligated to provide accounting, legally authorized, or otherwise qualifying services. If legal or technical advice is required, an expert should be contacted.

Any copying, duplication, or distribution of any portion of this book, whether electronic or written, is prohibited. Documentation and preservation of this publication are forbidden, and preservation of this document is only permitted with the author's explicit consent. Intellectual property rights are reserved.

The consumer takes full responsibility for any liability arising from the use or violation of any laws, procedures, or directions included herein, whether due to inattention or otherwise. The publisher will not be held responsible for any damages, mistakes, or monetary loss suffered as a consequence of the information provided herein, whether directly or indirectly. The writer owns the copyrights.

This material is provided purely for educational purposes and is therefore universal. The data is given without any kind of assurance or agreement. The trademarks are used without the trademark owner's permission or support. The trademarks and labels mentioned in this book belong to their respective owners, and this material is in no way affiliated with them

Table of Contents

Introduction

Eat disorders are mental illnesses characterized by aberrant eating practices that have a detrimental impact on the physical or mental health of the individual suffering from them. At any one moment, only one eating problem may be identified and treated. The following types of eating disorders are recognized: binge eating disorder, in which the afflicted consumes a large amount of food in a short period of time; anorexia nervosa, in which the afflicted has an intense fear of gaining weight and restricts food or over exercises to manage this fear; bulimia nervosa, in which the afflicted consumes a large amount of food (bingeing) and then attempts to rid themselves People who suffer from eating disorders are more likely than the general population to suffer from anxiety disorders, depression, and drug misuse. Obesity is not included in this list of disorders.

The reasons of eating disorders are not completely understood, while it seems that both biological and environmental factors have a role. It is claimed that the cultural idealization of thinness contributes to the development of various eating disorders. Individuals who have been sexually abused are also more prone to acquire eating problems than the general population. In certain cases, such as pica and rumination disorder, persons with intellectual impairments are more likely to suffer from these conditions.

Many eating problems may be successfully treated with medication. A variety of treatments are available, depending on the problem. These include counselling, nutritional guidance, minimizing excessive activity, and lessening attempts to remove food. Medications may be used to alleviate some of the symptoms associated with the condition. The requirement for hospitalization may be necessary in more extreme circumstances. Approximately 70% of persons with anorexia and 50% of those with bulimia recover within five years after being diagnosed with the disorder.

Recovery from binge eating disorder is less certain and is considered to be between 20 percent and 60 percent of the population. In both anorexia and bulimia, the risk of mortality is increased. Prevalence estimates for eating disorders are very variable, reflecting disparities in gender, age, and culture, as well as differences in the diagnostic and measuring methodologies used to make the determination. Anorexia affects around 0.4 percent of young women in the industrialized world, whereas bulimia affects approximately 1.3 percent of young women in the same year. On an annual basis, about 1.6 percent of females and 0.8 percent of males are affected by binge eating disorder According to one study, the percentage of women who will suffer from anorexia at some time in their life may be as high as 4 percent, whereas the percentage of women who will suffer from bulimia and binge eating disorders may be as low as 2 percent. In less developed nations, the prevalence of eating disorders seems to be lower. Females suffer from anorexia and bulimia at a rate that is about 10 times greater than that of men. Eating disorders often manifest themselves throughout late childhood to early adulthood. It is unclear what the prevalence of other eating disorders is. **Let's Get Started!**

Chapter No.01

Eating Disorders

In addition to severe and persistent disturbances in eating behaviours, eating disorders are characterized by painful thoughts and feelings that accompany the eating behaviour disruption. They may be life-threatening disorders that impair physical, psychological, and social functioning, among other things. Anorexia nervosa, bulimia nervosa, binge eating disorder, avoidant restricted food intake disorder, and other specified feeding and eating disorder, pica, and rumination disorder are all examples of eating disorders. Eating disorders, when considered as a group, impact up to 5% of the population, with the majority of cases occurring throughout adolescence and early adulthood. Anorexia Nervosa and Bulimia Nervosa are two disorders that are more frequent in women than in men, although they may afflict anyone of any age and are not limited to females or males. Eating disorders are often connected with preoccupations with food, weight, or form, as well as with anxiety about consuming and the repercussions of eating specific foods, according to the National Institute of Health.

Consumption patterns related with eating disorders include restricted eating or avoidance of certain foods, binge eating, purging via vomiting or laxative usage, and obsessive exercise, among others. These behaviours may become compelled in ways that seem to be similar to those associated with addiction. At any one moment, eating disorders affect several million individuals, the majority of whom are females between the ages of 12 and 35. A person suffering from an eating disorder is classified as having one of three types: anorexia nervosa, bulimia nervosa, or binge eating disorder.

Eating disorders often occur in conjunction with other mental diseases, the most prevalent of which are mood and anxiety disorders, obsessive compulsive disorder, and alcohol and drug misuse issues. Despite the fact that evidence shows that genes and heredity play a role in why certain individuals are at greater risk for eating disorders, eating disorders may affect people who do not have a family history of the problem. Psychological, behavioural, dietary, and other medical issues should all be addressed throughout treatment. Various potentially deadly illnesses include cardiac and gastrointestinal issues, as well as other complications of starvation or purging habits. The presence of ambivalence about therapy, denial of the existence of an eating or weight issue, or concern about altering eating habits are all not unusual. Those suffering from eating disorders, on the other hand, may regain control of their eating habits as well as their emotional and psychological well-being with adequate medical treatment.

1.1 Types of Eating Disorders

1.1.1 Anorexia Nervosa

Dietary restriction and weight loss are hallmarks of anorexia nervosa, which results in abnormally low weight for one's height and age. It is important to note that anorexia has the greatest death rate of any mental diagnosis other than opioid use disorder, and that it may be a life-threatening illness. With anorexia nervosa, the body mass index (BMI), which measures weight in relation to height, is often less than 18.5 in an adult person.

Those who suffer from anorexia nervosa engage in dieting because they are terrified of gaining weight or becoming obese. Despite the fact that some persons with anorexia claim to desire and are attempting to gain weight, their conduct does not correspond to their stated intentions. For example, they may only consume tiny quantities of low-calorie items while engaging in vigorous physical activity. Some people who suffer from anorexia nervosa also binge eat and purge on a regular basis, either via vomiting or the overuse of laxatives.

Anorexia nervosa may be classified into two subtypes:

- The limiting type, in which people lose weight largely by dieting, fasting, or severe exercise, is also known as the restrictive type.
- the binge-eating/purging kind, in which individuals engage in occasional binge eating and/or purging behaviours in addition to regular binge eating and/or purging behaviours.

Symptoms of Anorexia Nervosa

- The cessation of menstrual periods
- Feeling dizzy or faint as a result of dehydration
- Hair and nails that are brittle
- Intolerance to the cold
- weakness and atrophy of the muscles
- Acid reflux and heartburn (in those who vomit)
- Severe constipation, bloating, and a feeling of being stuffed after meals
- Osteoporosis and osteopenia are both conditions caused by excessive activity, and stress fractures are a complication of both (thinning of the bones)

Depression, anger, anxiety, poor focus, and exhaustion are all symptoms of bipolar disorder. Patients who vomit or use laxatives are more likely to have serious medical issues, which may be life-threatening. These complications include cardiac rhythm irregularities (particularly in those who vomit or use laxatives), renal difficulties, and seizures.

In order to treat anorexia nervosa, it is necessary to assist people who are afflicted in reestablishing appropriate eating and weight management practices as well as restoring their weight. Co-occurring mental and medical disorders should be evaluated and treated as part of the treatment strategy. The dietary plan should be focused on assisting people in overcoming their fear of eating and encouraging them to consume a diverse and balanced variety of foods with varying calorie densities over the course of many regularly spaced meals. The most successful therapies for teenagers entail assisting parents in providing assistance and monitoring their child's mealtimes. In addition to weight and eating habits, addressing body dissatisfaction is crucial, although it frequently takes longer to rectify than the former.

Admission to an inpatient or residential behavioural specialty program may be recommended in the event of severe anorexia nervosa when outpatient therapy has failed to provide satisfactory results. Though most specialty programs are successful in restoring weight and returning eating habits to normal, the risk of recurrence in the first year after program completion remains high.

1.2   Bulimia Nervosa

Individuals suffering from bulimia nervosa often cycle between dieting, or eating only low-calorie "safe meals," and binge eating high-calorie items that are "forbidden." Binge eating is described as consuming a big quantity of food in a short period of time while feeling a lack of control over what or how much one is eating. It is connected with a sense of loss of control over what and how much one is eating. Binge behaviour is often hidden and accompanied by emotions of guilt or humiliation, according to the experts. Binges may be quite enormous, and food is often devoured quickly, past the point of fullness, resulting in nausea and discomfort.

Binge eating occurs at least once a week, and it is usually followed by what are known as "compensatory behaviours" in order to avoid weight gain. Fasting, vomiting, laxative abuse, and obsessive exercise are all examples of compulsive behaviours. Persons suffering from bulimia nervosa, like those suffering from anorexia nervosa, are overly obsessed with ideas about food, weight, or form, which have a negative influence on their self-worth and have a disproportionate impact on it.

Patients with bulimia nervosa may be of any weight, from slightly underweight to average weight to overweight or obese. They are deemed to have anorexia nervosa binge-eating/purging type, rather than bulimia nervosa, if they are underweight, as opposed to being overweight. Family members or friends may be unaware that a person has bulimia nervosa because the individual does not seem to be underweight and because the person's activities are disguised and may go undetected by people who are close to him or her. The following are examples of indicators that someone may be suffering from bulimia nervosa:

- Frequent visits to the restroom immediately after meals
- Large quantities of food vanishing or going missing for no apparent reason; empty wrappers and food containers;
- Sore throat that lasts a long time
- A swelling of the salivary glands in the cheeks is another symptom.
- Gastric acid erosion causes dental decay, which results in the erosion of tooth enamel.
- Acid reflux and gastro esophageal reflux disease
- Misuse of laxatives or diet pills
- Unexplained diarrhea that occurs on a regular basis
- Excessive use of diuretics (water pills)
- Experiencing dizziness or fainting due to dehydration as a consequence of excessive purging actions

Complications of binge eating disorder, such as esophageal rips and stomach rupture, as well as hazardous cardiac rhythms, are uncommon but may be deadly in certain cases. Medical monitoring is critical in the treatment of severe bulimia nervosa because it allows doctors to recognize and treat any potential issues that may arise.

Outpatient cognitive behavioural therapy for bulimia nervosa is the treatment having the most evidence to support its effectiveness. It assists patients in normalizing their eating habit as well as managing thoughts and emotions that contribute to the disorder's progression. Antidepressants may also be beneficial in reducing the desire to overindulge and vomit. Binge Eating Disorder is a kind of eating disorder that occurs when a person consumes an excessive amount of food in a short period of time. People who suffer from binge eating disorder, like those who suffer from bulimia nervosa, have bouts of binge eating in which they consume huge amounts of food in a short period of time, feel a lack of control over their eating, and are upset as a result of their binge behaviour. However, unlike those suffering from bulimia nervosa, they do not engage in compensatory behaviours such as producing vomiting, fasting, exercising, or abusing laxatives on a regular basis in order to get rid of the food. Bulking up on food is a chronic condition that may lead to major health consequences, such as obesity and diabetes, as well as hypertension and cardiovascular disease. The presence of frequent binges (at least once a week for three months) accompanied with a sensation of loss of control, as well as three or more of the following characteristics, is required for the diagnosis of binge eating disorder:

- Consuming food at a faster rate than usual
- Consuming food till one is uncomfortably full
- Consuming excessive quantities of food despite the fact that one is not hungry
- Eating alone because one is embarrassed by the amount of food one is consuming
- Feeling ashamed with oneself, dejected, or very guilty as a result of the experience

In the same way that bulimia nervosa is treated, cognitive behavioural psychotherapy for binge eating is the most effective treatment for binge eating disorder. Interpersonal therapy, as well as many antidepressant drugs, have all been found to be useful in the treatment of depression.

1.3 Feeding and Eating Disorders

Eat disorders or eating behaviour problems that cause distress and impede familial, social, or occupational function but do not fall into any of the other diagnostic categories described below are included in this diagnostic category. Occasionally, this is due to a lack of compliance with the diagnostic threshold (for example, the frequency of binges in bulimia or bulimia nervosa) or a failure to fulfil the weight criterion for the diagnosis of anorexia nervosa in rare situations.

"Atypical anorexia nervosa" is an example of a specific feeding and eating disorder that is not included here. In this category are individuals who, although they may have lost significant amounts of weight and exhibited behaviours and a high level of fear of being fat that are consistent with anorexia nervosa, are not yet considered underweight according to their BMI because their starting weight was above average. Because the rate at which people lose weight is associated with the likelihood of developing medical complications, people who lose a significant amount of weight quickly by engaging in extreme weight control behaviours may be at increased risk of developing medical complications, even if their weight appears normal or above average.

1.4   Avoidant Restrictive Food Intake Disorder

Arrested/restricted food intake disorder (ARFID) is a newly described eating disorder that is characterized by a disruption in eating that results in a chronic inability to achieve nutritional requirements and an intense preference for fussy foods. Food avoidance or a restricted food repertoire may be caused by one or more of the following factors in ARFID:

- A lack of interest in eating or food, as well as a lack of desire
- Food avoidance to extremes depending on sensory aspects of foods, such as texture, look, colour, and smell.
- Fear of choking; nausea; vomiting; constipation; an allergic response; and other concerns about the effects of eating when a substantial negative event occurs, such as choking or food poisoning, the condition may develop as a result of the avoidance of a growing number of foods over a period of time.

In order to be diagnosed with ARFID, it is necessary that eating disorders be connected with one or more of the following factors:

- Significant reduction in body weight (or failure to achieve expected weight gain in children).
- Nutrient deficit of significant magnitude
- The need for a feeding tube or oral nutritional supplements in order to ensure adequate nutrient intake.
- Interference with the capacity to operate socially (such as inability to eat with others).

The effect on physical and psychological health, as well as the degree of starvation, might be comparable to that experienced by those suffering from anorexia nervosa. People who suffer from ARFID, on the other hand, do not have excessive worries about their body weight or form, and the illness is separate from anorexia nervosa or bulimia nervosa, which are both eating disorders. Individuals with autism spectrum condition often exhibit rigid eating patterns and sensory sensitivity, although they do not always result in the amount of impairment necessary for a diagnosis of avoidant/restrictive food intake disorder. Dietary restrictions due to a shortage of food availability; appropriate dieting; cultural customs such as religious fasting; or developmentally typical habits such as fussy eaters in toddlers are excluded from the definition of ARFID.

When it comes to food avoidance or limitation, it is most frequent in infancy or early childhood, and it may last until maturity. It, on the other hand, may begin at any age. ARFID may have a negative influence on families, regardless of the age of the individual afflicted. It can cause higher stress during mealtimes and other social eating settings.

In order to treat ARFID, each patient must have a specific treatment plan that may include numerous professionals, including a mental health professional, a registered dietitian nutritionist, and others.

1.5   Pica

Pica is a kind of eating problem in which a person consumes items that are not food and have no nutritional value on a regular basis. The conduct has persisted for at least one month and is serious enough to necessitate seeking medical assistance for the individual. Paper, paint chips, soap, fabric, hair, thread, chalk, metal, stones, charcoal or coal, and clay are some of the more common items that people consume, depending on their age and available resources. Individuals who suffer from pica do not often have a strong aversion to any particular foods.

The conduct is improper for the individual's developmental stage and does not correspond to a culturally recognized practice. It is not acceptable. Pica may manifest itself at any stage of life, including infancy, adolescence, and adults, however it is most frequent in childhood. Children under the age of two are not diagnosed with it. For youngsters under the age of two, putting little items in their mouths is a typical aspect of their development. Pica is most often associated with autism spectrum disorder and intellectual handicap, however it may also occur in children who are otherwise well developing.

A person who has been diagnosed with pica is at danger of developing intestinal obstructions or experiencing harmful consequences from the drugs they ingest (e.g. lead in paint chips). Pica treatment consists of checking for nutritional inadequacies and, if necessary, treating such deficiencies. Behavior therapies used to treat pica may involve shifting the individual's attention away from nonfood objects and praising them for putting nonfood items aside or avoiding them altogether.

1.5   Rumination Disorder

It is characterized by the frequent regurgitation and re-chewing of food after eating, in which swallowed food is taken back up into the mouth willingly and re-chewed and swallowed, or spit out, by the person suffering from the disease. Rumination disorder may manifest itself in infancy, youth, adolescence, or maturity. Rumination disorder is a kind of anxiety illness. The following behaviours must be seen in order to fulfil the diagnosis:

- When it occurs regularly over the course of at least one month, it is considered severe.
- Not be the result of a gastrointestinal or medical condition
- Does not occur in conjunction with any of the other behavioural eating disorders indicated above.
- In addition to mental problems (e.g., intellectual impairment), ruminating may occur in other conditions as well; however, the severity of the ruminating must be severe enough to demand distinct professional attention in order to be diagnosed.

1.6 Causes of Eating Disorder

Many variables, according to experts, may contribute to the development of eating disorders. Genetics is one of these topics. Studies of twins and adoptions involving twins who were separated at birth and adopted by different families give some indication that eating disorders may be passed down through the family. According to the findings of this sort of study, if one twin has an eating problem, the other twin has a 50 percent chance of having one as well, according to the findings.

Another factor is a person's personality qualities. The personality qualities of neuroticism, perfectionism, and impulsivity in particular are three characteristics that are often associated with an increased risk of having an eating problem. Other possible explanations include perceived social pressures to be thin, cultural preferences for thinness, and exposure to media that promotes such ideals of thinness and health. According to the research findings, some eating disorders are almost non-existent among cultures that have not been exposed to Western standards of thinness and body shape.

Having said that, thinness ideals that are culturally acceptable are highly prevalent in many parts of the globe. Despite this, only a small number of people develop an eating problem in various nations. As a result, they are most likely the result of a combination of causes. The development of eating disorders may also be influenced by variations in brain anatomy and biology, according to current theories advanced by scientists and researchers. Particularly important may be the amounts of the neurotransmitters serotonin and dopamine in the brain. There are a variety of reasons that might contribute to eating disorders. Genetics, brain biology, personality characteristics, and cultural standards are examples of such factors.

Chapter No. 02

Factors of Eating Disorder on Human Life

Eating disorders affect women at a higher rate than males, according to the National Eating Disorders Association. Aside from genetic and environmental variables, there are other factors such as social and environmental factors that may raise your chance of having an eating problem. These include:

- age
- ancestors and forefathers
- dieting to an extreme degree
- the state of one's mental health
- changes in one's life
- participation in extracurricular activities

2.1   Age
Eating disorders may develop at any age, although they are more frequent in adolescents and early twenties, despite the fact that they can occur at any age.

2.2   Ancestors and forefathers
An individual's vulnerability to having an eating problem may be influenced by their genetic makeup. In accordance with the Mayo Clinic, those who have

first-degree relatives who suffer from an eating problem are more likely to suffer from the disease themselves.

2.3   Excessive dieting is harmful

Weight reduction is often accompanied with positive reinforcement. Eating more severely in order to satisfy your desire for affirmation might result in an eating problem.

2.4   Psychological health

If you have an eating disorder, it is possible that you have an underlying psychological or mental health issue that is contributing to your condition. These issues might include the following:

- a poor sense of self-worth
- anxiety
- depression
- The condition known as Obsessive-Compulsive Disorder
- partnerships that are in disarray
- a tendency to act on the spur of the moment

2.5   Transitions in one's life

Certain events and changes in one's life might generate emotional pain and worry, which can increase one's risk of developing an eating problem. Especially if you've suffered with an eating issue in the past, this is important to remember. Moving, changing employment, the termination of a relationship, or the loss of a loved one are all examples of transitional events. Abuse, sexual assault, and incest are all factors that might contribute to an eating problem.

2.6 Extracurricular activities

Participating in sports teams or artistic organizations puts you at a higher chance of being a victim. All members of any community that is driven by looks as a marker of social standing, including sports, actresses, dancers, models, and television celebrities, are subject to the same rules as everyone else. The weight reduction encouragement provided by coaches, parents, and other experts in these fields may unintentionally encourage eating disorders.

2.7 Percentage of teens suffer from eating disorders

Teenagers are particularly vulnerable to eating disorders because of the hormonal changes that occur throughout puberty, as well as societal pressure to seem attractive or slim. It is typical for your adolescent to experience these changes, and he or she may engage in bad eating behaviours just on occasion. In contrast, if your adolescent begins to obsess about their weight, looks, or diet, or begins to eat excessively or insufficiently on a continuous basis, they may be developing an eating disorder. In addition, abnormal weight loss or increase may be a symptom of an eating problem, particularly if your adolescent often makes disparaging remarks about their body or perceived size.

If you have reason to believe your adolescent is suffering from an eating problem, be forthright and honest about your worries. If they feel safe sharing their problems with you, be compassionate and attentive to their needs. In addition, take them to visit a doctor, counsellor, or therapist to address any social or emotional problems that may be contributing to their condition.

2.8   Do eating problems impact males as well as women?

Women are more likely than males to suffer from eating problems, but guys are not exempt. According to research from Trusted Source, males who suffer from eating disorders are underdiagnosed and undertreated as well. Even when they display symptoms that are comparable to (or even the same as) those of a woman, men are less likely to be diagnosed with an eating problem. Some males suffer from a disorder known as muscle dysmorphia, which is characterized by an intense desire to gain muscle mass. While the majority of women who suffer from eating disorders seek to reduce weight and become thinner, the majority of men who suffer from eating disorders believe they are too tiny and wish to gain weight or build muscle mass. They may participate in potentially risky actions, such as the usage of steroids, and they may also use other forms of medicines in order to gain muscle bulk more rapidly.

A growing body of evidence shows that many young males with eating problems do not seek treatment because they see them as stereotypically feminine diseases.

2.9   Complications

Eating disorders are associated with a broad range of problems, some of which are life-threatening. Because eating disorders are severe and long-lasting, the likelihood of experiencing major problems increases. These complications include:

- Severe health-related issues
- Depression and anxiety are two of the most common ailments.
- Suicidal thoughts or actions are not uncommon.
- Issues pertaining to growth and development
- Problems in social and interpersonal relationships
- Substance abuse and dependence problems
- Concerns about work and school
- Death

2.10 Prevention

In spite of the fact that there is no sure-fire strategy to avoid eating disorders, the following measures may help your kid establish good eating habits:

- Avoid dieting in the presence of your youngster. The way a family eats may have an impact on the connections that children form with food. Eating meals together provides you the chance to educate your kid about the dangers of dieting while also encouraging him or her to consume a nutritious diet in moderate quantities.

- Have a conversation with your youngster. As an example, there are various websites that promote potentially harmful notions, such as the concept that anorexia is a lifestyle choice rather than an eating disorder, rather than an eating disorder. If your kid has any misconceptions about healthy eating, it is critical that you address them and speak to them about the dangers of making poor food choices.

- Encourage and reinforce a positive body image in your kid, no matter what his or her physical appearance is. Talk to your youngster about his or her self-image and reassure him or her that body forms might differ. Avoid making negative comments about your own physique in front of your youngster. Messages of acceptance and respect may aid in the development of good self-esteem and resilience in youngsters, which will help them navigate the difficult years of adolescence.

- Enlist the assistance of your child's physician. Doctors may be able to detect early signs of an eating issue in children during routine well-child checkups. During normal medical checkups, for example, they might ask youngsters questions about their eating habits and their contentment with their looks. Checks of height and weight percentiles as well as body mass index should be performed at these appointments, since these measurements may notify you and your child's doctor to any noteworthy changes.

If you have a family member or friend who seems to be suffering from an eating problem, you should consider discussing your concerns with him or her regarding his or her well-being. Despite the fact that you may not be able to prevent an eating problem from forming, showing compassion to the individual may inspire them to seek help.

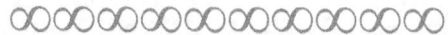

Chapter No. 03

Treatment of Eating Disorder

Treatment for an eating disorder is dependent on the specific disorder and symptoms you are experiencing. A combination of psychological therapy (psychotherapy), nutrition education, medical monitoring, and, on occasion, medications is used to treat the condition.

Eating disorder treatment also entails addressing any other health issues that have arisen as a result of the eating disorder, which can be serious or even life-threatening if left untreated for an extended period of time. It is possible that you will require hospitalization or another type of inpatient program if you're eating disorder does not improve with standard treatment or if it is causing health problems. Incorporating a systematic approach to eating disorder treatment can assist you in managing symptoms, returning to a healthy weight, and maintaining both your physical and mental health.

3.1 Where to Start?

Regardless of whether you begin by consulting with your primary care provider or a mental health professional, you will almost certainly benefit from being referred to a team of professionals who are trained in eating disorder treatment and recovery. Members of your treatment team may include the following individuals:

- **A mental health professional**, such as a psychologist, who will provide psychological therapy to the patient. When it comes to medication prescription and management, you may want to consult with a psychiatrist. Some psychiatrists also provide psychological therapy as an additional service.
- **A registered dietitian** who will educate participants on nutrition and meal planning topics.
- **Treatment for health or dental problems** that arise as a result of your eating disorder can be obtained from medical or dental specialists.
- **Your partner, parents, or other members of your family**. Parents should be actively involved in the treatment of their children who are still living at home, and they should be able to supervise meals.

It is preferable if everyone involved in your treatment is aware of your progress so that any necessary adjustments can be made to your treatment. Managing an eating disorder can be a difficult task over an extended period of time. Even if you're eating disorder and associated health problems are under control, you may need to continue seeing members of your treatment team on a regular basis.

3.2 Putting together a treatment strategy

You and your treatment team will work together to determine your needs and develop goals and guidelines for your treatment. Your treatment team collaborates with you in order to:

- Put together a treatment strategy. This includes developing a treatment strategy for your eating disorder as well as setting treatment objectives. It also makes it clear what you should do if you are unable to follow through with your plan.
- Take care of any physical complications. Health and medical problems that arise as a result of your eating disorder are closely monitored and addressed by your treatment team.
- Identify available resources. Your treatment team can assist you in determining what resources are available in your area to assist you in achieving your objectives.
- Identify treatment options that are within your budget. It can be expensive to receive treatment for an eating disorder in a hospital or an outpatient program, and your insurance may not cover the entire cost of your care. Financial issues and concerns should be discussed with your treatment team; treatment should not be

avoided because of the possibility of financial hardship.

3.3 Psychological therapy

When it comes to eating disorder treatment, psychological therapy is by far the most important component. Visiting a psychologist or another mental health professional on a regular basis is required.

Therapy can last anywhere from a few months to several years. It can assist you in the following ways:

- Establish a routine for your eating habits and reach a healthy weight.
- Replace unhealthy habits with more beneficial ones.
- Learn how to keep track of your food intake and your moods.
- Improve your problem-solving abilities.
- Investigate healthy coping mechanisms for dealing with stressful situations.
- Make your interpersonal relationships better.
- Make your mood better.

Treatment may include a combination of different types of therapy, including, but not limited to:

- **Cognitive behavioural therapy** (also known as CBT). An eating disorder is treated with this type of psychotherapy, which focuses on the behaviours, thoughts, and feelings that are associated with it. In addition to assisting you in developing healthy eating habits, it also assists you in learning to recognize and change distorted thoughts that contribute to eating disorder behaviours.

- **Therapy that is centered on the family**. The goal of this therapy is to teach family members how to assist you in re-establishing healthy eating patterns and attaining a healthy weight until you are able to do so on your own. This type of therapy can be particularly beneficial for parents who are learning how to assist a teen suffering from an eating disorder.
- **Cognitive behavioural therapy** in a group setting. An eating disorder support group consists of people who have been diagnosed with an eating disorder who meet with a psychologist or another mental health professional on a regular basis. In addition to helping you address your eating disorder-related thoughts, feelings, and behaviours, it can also help you learn skills to manage your symptoms and reestablish healthy eating patterns.

Some homework assignments may be assigned by your psychologist or other mental health professional, such as keeping a food journal to review in therapy sessions and identifying triggers that lead to bingeing or purging, or engaging in other unhealthy eating behaviours.

3.4   Nutritional counselling and education

Registered dietitians and other professionals who are involved in your treatment can assist you in better understanding you're eating disorder and in developing a plan to achieve and maintain healthy eating habits in the long term. The following may be the objectives of nutrition education:

- Make an effort to maintain a healthy weight.
- Gain an understanding of how nutrition affects your body, including recognizing how you're eating disorder contributes to nutrition issues and physical issues.
- Put your meal planning skills to the test.
- Establish regular eating patterns — three meals a day, plus regular snacks — and stick with them.
- Take preventative measures to avoid dieting or bingeing.
- Resolve any health issues that have arisen as a result of malnutrition or obesity

3.5   Medications for the treatment of eating disorders

An eating disorder cannot be cured with medication. When used in conjunction with psychological therapy, they are the most effective. Antidepressants are the most commonly prescribed medications for the treatment of eating disorders that involve binge-eating or purging behaviours, but other medications may also be prescribed depending on the circumstances. If you suffer from bulimia or binge-eating disorder, you may find that taking an antidepressant is particularly beneficial. Antidepressants can also help to alleviate the symptoms of depression or anxiety, which are frequently experienced by people who suffer from eating disorders. You may also require medication to treat physical health problems that have arisen as a result of your eating disorder.

3.6 Admission to a psychiatric facility for eating disorders

If you have serious physical or mental health problems, or if you have anorexia and are unable to eat or gain weight, you may need to be admitted to a hospital for treatment. Physical health problems that are severe or life-threatening that occur as a result of anorexia should be treated as a medical emergency. Most of the time, the most important goal of hospitalization is to stabilize acute medical symptoms by initiating the process of returning to a normal eating and weight routine. The majority of eating disorders and weight restoration procedures are performed in an outpatient setting.

3.7 Programs for inpatient day treatment in hospitals

In most cases, day treatment programs are highly structured and require attendance for a number of hours each day, several days a week. Medical care, group, individual, and family therapy, structured eating sessions, and nutrition education are all possible components of day treatment.

3.8 Treatment for eating disorders in a residential setting

Residential treatment is a type of treatment in which you temporarily relocate to an eating disorder treatment facility. A residential treatment program may be necessary if you require long-term care for your eating disorder or if you have been admitted to the hospital on a number of occasions but have not seen any improvement in your mental or physical health.

3.9 Treatment for health problems that are ongoing

Eating disorders can cause serious health problems related to inadequate nutrition, overeating, bingeing and other factors. The type of health problems caused by eating disorders depends on the type and severity of the eating disorder. In many cases, problems caused by an eating disorder require ongoing treatment and monitoring.

Health problems linked to eating disorders may include:

- Electrolyte imbalances, which can interfere with the functioning of your muscles, heart and nerves
- Heart problems and high blood pressure
- Digestive difficulties
- Nutrient deficiencies
- Dental cavities and degradation of the surface of your teeth from recurrent vomiting (bulimia) (bulimia)
- Low bone density (osteoporosis) as a consequence of irregular or nonexistent menstruation or long-term starvation (anorexia) (anorexia)
- Stunted development induced by insufficient nutrition (anorexia) (anorexia)
- Mental health issues such as depression, anxiety, obsessive-compulsive disorder or drug addiction
- Lack of menstruation and issues with infertility and pregnancy

Take an active part

You are the most crucial part of your treatment team. For effective therapy, you need to be actively engaged in your treatment and so do your family members and other loved ones. Your treatment team can give education and advise you where to get further information and assistance.

There's a lot of misinformation regarding eating disorders on the web, so heed your treatment team's recommendations and obtain ideas on credible websites to learn more about your eating problem. Examples of useful websites include the National Eating Disorders Association (NEDA), as well as Families Empowered and Supporting Treatment of Eating Disorders (F.E.A.S.T.).

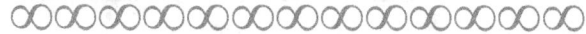

Chapter No. 04

Health

4.1 Health

It is vital to maintain overall physical, mental, social, and spiritual well-being in order to preserve the body to the maximum degree feasible by daily counselling and preventive activities to reduce the likelihood of illness. When it comes to being happy, one's health has a huge influence on one's capacity to do so. Many people suffer from illnesses, but being in excellent health enables them to fight the diseases and maintain physical fitness, enabling them to feel comfortable and enjoy life as much as any other normal person would.

4.2 The Importance of Good Health in a Person's Daily Life

Health is described as the body's ability to carry out its duties and burn calories effectively, as well as its ability to adapt to changes in the physical, mental, and social environments in which it finds itself.

Having good health is essential for carrying out one's daily duties in the most efficient and effective manner possible. The body of a person must be free of sicknesses in all sections of his or her body, as well as free of sickness in all of his or her bodily membranes, in order to be in excellent physical health. If we are talking about mental and social health, the ability of a person to carry out social tasks that have been given to him without fault or error is a good sign of how healthy they are. No one can disagree that good health is very vital in one's day-to-day interactions with others. In this book, we will cover a number of important issues that will clearly clarify the relevance of health in our lives as well as how we might obtain better health.

In addition to people, the presence of disease among its members has an influence on society as a whole since the productivity of these patients' falls and they become dependent on the rest of society. A healthy population in a society translates into a population of productive people who have the strength and ability to contribute to their communities and help those in need. People's lives are made more meaningful by their health since it helps them to avoid the high costs of medical treatment while also eliminating the bother of having to attend hospitals. In the viewpoint of a healthy person who is far away from the illness, money is saved that would have otherwise been spent on the ailment if the person had ignored his or her own health and chosen to ignore the illness. Because of this, it is often said. According to what you can see, many governments that are prone to the development of diseases and illnesses among their inhabitants spend a large percentage of their budgets on the procurement of medications in order to battle these epidemics and illnesses. You will also discover governments and cultures that are worried about the safety of their inhabitants and are focused on areas such as preventative medicine and health counselling to achieve this goal.

A healthy person may be seen enjoying his or her life, building relationships with other people, and demonstrating love, compassion, and connectedness to those around him or her. A person must also consider a wide range of concerns and behaviours throughout his or her life in order to avoid diseases that interfere with his or her everyday activities and to acknowledge that illness may be one of the many difficulties to which he or she is confronted.

4.3   Health and Medical Psychology

Human health psychology is a discipline within psychological science that investigates the ways in which variables such as biology, psychology, behaviour and social factors influence an individual's health and well-being. Along with the term "health psychology," other ideas such as "medical psychology" and "behavioural medicine" are frequently used interchangeably with the term "health psychology."

Various factors may have an influence on one's health and well-being, and there is no one cause for this effect.

There is a high prevalence of contagious and hereditary illness, but there are also behavioural and psychological factors that impact overall physical well-being and the incidence of various medical conditions. It is the goal of health psychology to promote and preserve good health, as well as to prevent and cure disease and illness-related conditions. Individuals' responses to sickness, as well as how they cope with and recover from illness, are all studied by health psychologists. It is the goal of some health psychologists' work to improve both the health-care system itself and the government's attitude to health-care policy.

Division 38 of the American Psychological Association is devoted to the study of health psychology and its applications. According to the division's mission statement, its primary goals are to gain a better understanding of health and illness, conduct research into the psychological factors that influence health, and contribute to the improvement of the health-care system and public health policies in the United States. Because of the continually changing nature of the healthcare business, the field of health psychology was formed in reaction to this in the 1970s. According to current statistics, people in the United States may expect to live for around 80 years on average, with chronic diseases accounting for the majority of deaths, many of which are linked to one's way of life. 2 Dealing with these changes in health may be made easier with the help of health psychology.

4.4   What Makes Health Psychology So Special

In part due to the fact that health psychology emphasizes the link between behaviour and health, it is well suited to assisting people in altering the behaviours that are damaging to their health and well-being. Applied study on how to prevent hazardous habits such as smoking and the exploration of creative strategies to promote healthy behaviours such as exercise, to mention a few examples, might be carried out by psychologists in this field.

Many people continue to engage in such behaviours, despite the fact that the majority of people recognize that consuming a high-sugar diet is detrimental to their health. This is true regardless of the possible short- and long-term consequences of their actions. Mental health professionals that specialize in health behaviour explore the psychological factors that influence people's health choices and look for ways that might motivate people into making better health decisions. Information on fatalities in the United States and the variables that lead to them is collected by the National Center for Health Statistics, an arm of the Centers for Disease Control and Prevention (CDC). In the United States, according to data trends over the last century, roughly half of all deaths may be traced back to behaviours or other risk factors that are mostly preventable.

According to the most recent Centers for Disease Control and Prevention study (2012), the incidence of mortality has decreased for all primary causes of death except suicide; life expectancy has reached an all-time high (78.8 years); and yet, approximately 83 Americans die from heart disease and stroke every hour in the United States. It is possible that more than a fifth of the deaths may have been averted. Mortality due to cancer remained in second place, followed by deaths due to chronic lower respiratory illnesses, such as chronic bronchitis; drug poisoning, especially overdoses; and fatal falls among the elderly rounded out the top five causes of death in this group.

4.5   Health Psychology: Current Issues and Perspectives

Health psychologists work with individuals, groups, communities, and organizations to reduce risk factors and improve overall health while also minimizing disease. They do research and provide services in a wide range of subjects, including the ones listed below.

- It is critical to reduce stress levels.
- Keeping one's weight under control
- Improve the nutritious content of your ordinary meals.

- Hospice care and grief counselling are also available.
- Preventing the occurrence of illness
- Recognizing the ramifications of sickness
- Increasing the efficiency with which recovery is accomplished
- Educating children on effective coping techniques

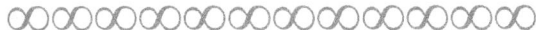

Chapter No. 05

Eating habits and behaviors

Food provides our bodies with the energy they need to perform properly. Traditions and culture are woven into the fabric of food. That eating may have an emotional component can be seen as follows: Changing one's eating habits may be quite difficult for many individuals. It's possible that you've been practicing harmful eating habits for a long time and aren't even aware of it. Alternatively, your behaviours have become ingrained in your daily routine, and you no longer give them any thought.

5.1 The Worst Eating Habits in the World

No one, not even dietitians, can eat correctly all of the time. When unhealthy habits become normal practice, however, they may lead to weight gain, high cholesterol, high blood pressure, and a variety of other possible health issues as a result of the consequences. So, what are the bad behaviours that are causing people to get into trouble? Here are the top ten blunders on our hit list, as well as tips on how to prevent them. How many are a regular part of your daily routine?

5.1.1 Inadequate Meal Preparation

The lack of "time," according to our readers, is one of the most significant obstacles to healthy eating. However, last-minute choices often result in trips to the drive-through and pizza delivery. It will save you money, calories, and time in the long run to spend a few minutes each week planning your weekly meals before you go grocery shopping for the week. Are you in a hurry? Tonight, try one of these nutritious, 20-minute meals >>

5.1.2 Excessive number of meals away from home

Restaurants and take-out will always serve up super-sized quantities, as well as higher calorie and salt counts than home cooking. Make an effort to make meals at home most nights of the week, and remember to follow our recommendations when you do go out to dinner.

5.1.3 There are much too many processed foods

Salty and greasy convenience meals that have been stripped of their nutritional value may be found everywhere. When possible, choose largely fresh and whole foods, and check labels to ensure that you are making the healthiest possible choices when you do decide to indulge in more heavily processed items. Get our 10 ideas on how to be a knowledgeable label reader by clicking here >>

5.1.4 Excessive use of added sugar

Sugar may be found in unexpected areas, such as whole grain cereals, salad dressings, sauces, and breads, in addition to the sweets, cookies, and soda that Americans currently consume in excess. Take stock of the entire amount of sugar in your diet and look for methods to reduce the number of empty calories you consume.

5.1.5 Consumption of food without consideration

We eat for a variety of reasons other than simply hunger. We eat when we're bored or weary or worried or happy or sad or anything else you can think of. Take a look at our suggestions for eating sensibly and for the right reasons.

5.1.6 Not Sharing a Meal with Others

The same way that eating mindlessly is associated with eating when preoccupied, overscheduled, or working several shifts. Shut off the television (and computer or mobile phone) during meals and try to sit down as a family for as many of them as you can throughout the day.

5.1.7 Eat on the Run

When you leave the home for a busy day without packing snacks or meals, you are setting yourself up for a diet catastrophe. You'll turn to foods that are overly processed, overly heavy, and overly detrimental to your waistline.

5.1.8 Portion Sizes

Even while you may believe you can judge portion sizes by eyeballing them, have you ever measured out your morning cereal, spoonful of peanut butter, or olive oil for cooking? Overindulging in portions (even while eating nutritious meals) might result in a calorie overload. Just go over it a couple times to get some perspective on the situation. Get our recommendations for the ideal portion sizes.

5.1.9 Excessive Consumption of Liquid Calories

Many people forget that calories from soda, juice, and other sugar-sweetened drinks must be taken into consideration. Replace high-calorie beverages with calorie-free alternatives such as water, unsweetened teas, and seltzer water. Do you dislike water? Try some of these low-calorie ways to spice things up >>

5.1.10 Not Consuming Enough Nutrients throughout the Day

Less isn't always better when it comes to fashion! Overeating later on (when you're weary and eager to eat everything in sight) is caused by not consuming enough calories during the day. This depletes energy levels, increases appetite, and causes weight gain. Spreading out calories throughout the day, beginning with a nutritious breakfast, can help you avoid overindulging in the afternoon and evening. Don't you wish there were more than 24 hours in a day so you could get more things done on your "to do" list? When it comes to juggling job and family life, this is the mindset of many people in the United States. As a consequence, we develop bad eating habits, such as shoveling food down our throats without taking the time to savior it. Here are some of the most egregious eating habits that we witness on a daily basis.

5.1.11 eating while staring at a computer screen

How many times have you tried to get your job done during your lunch hour while eating in front of your computer and failed? You wind up eating aimlessly and without even recognizing how much you've consumed. People are more likely to overeat as a result of this. Even worse, our children are modelling their eating patterns after ours. Consider this: do your children like eating in front of the television at night or when they are completing their homework? Solve it by taking a break from the computer, clearing your head, and enjoying your meal.

5.1.12 Walking and munching

I've seen this really brilliant dance hundreds of times, particularly when wandering around New York City with my friends. Pizza is the most common meal purchased on the street. Let's face it, that's hardly the ideal way to enjoy the tastiest pizza on the planet! Solution: Find a beautiful park or bench where you can sit and enjoy your meal while taking in the beautiful scenery.

5.1.13 Meal skipping

Some people find themselves unable to eat because they are too busy. They rush out of the house in the morning, attend meetings throughout the afternoon, and before you know it, its dinner time! According to research, skipping meals is associated with overeating at the following meal. You'll also notice that your energy levels aren't at their peak as a result of not getting enough calories throughout the day. Improve your planning skills and you'll be in good shape. Preparing a quick breakfast at your fingertips and keeping easy-to-eat snacks on hand for when you're in a hurry are essential.

5.1.14 consuming meal replacements

Healthy individuals are not required to consume meal replacements on a regular basis. Aside from being unappealing to the taste buds, these man-made concoctions lack the nutritional value that comes from real food. Whole foods contain phytonutrients, which are plant chemicals that can aid in the fight against or prevention of disease; however, the majority of these nutrients are not found in liquid meal replacements.

Solution: Keep the liquid supplements on hand in case of an actual emergency. Instead, pack a brown bag lunch for a quick and easy lunch in the morning.

5.1.15 forgetting to consume alcohol

Proper hydration can assist in maintaining energy levels throughout the day. Many people are so preoccupied with their jobs that they forget to drink enough water or other liquids. They become fatigued, have a headache, and are generally grumpy as a result.

5.2   Bad Eating Habits Can Be Changed

The majority of people are creatures of habit. We regularly shop at the same grocery store, cook the same meals time and time again, and conduct our lives according to our own set of established habits. In order to make significant progress in eating better and losing weight, you must alter your eating patterns and begin to think about nutrition and lifestyle in a new light.

The difficulty is that we get so used to our routines that it becomes difficult to break free of those old behaviours. A fear of the unknown or trying something new keeps many people from changing their diets, according to Dr. John Foreyt of the Baylor College of Medicine Behavioral Medicine Research Center. "Many people are sceptical about changing their diets because they have grown accustomed to eating or drinking the same foods, and there is a fear of the unknown or trying something new," he says.

Even when you have a strong desire to change, old habits are difficult to break.

The author of Foreyt's book states that habits become automatic, learnt actions over time, and that they are stronger than the new habits that you are attempting to introduce into your life. Even people who are successful in changing their unhealthy eating habits might simply revert to their old patterns when faced with a stressful situation. When you're feeling weak or vulnerable, your natural reflexes typically take precedence over your best interests. As Foreyt explains, "Everything might be going swimmingly until you reach a hard patch and begin experiencing sensations of boredom, loneliness, sadness, or... any form of stress." Foreyt believes that overcoming poor diet and physical activity habits involves a three-pronged approach:

- Being conscious of the harmful behaviours that you wish to break.
- Discovering the underlying causes of these behaviours.
- Determining how you'll gradually shift from your current unhealthy diet and activity routines to new, better ones.

These six stages will assist you in letting go of your old, harmful behaviours and replacing them with new, healthier ones:

5.2.1 Start with little steps

Making simple modifications to your food and lifestyle may have a significant impact on your health and ability to lose weight. Here are some recommendations from the experts:

- Make a point of eating a healthy breakfast every day.
- Get at least 8 hours of sleep every night, since weariness may contribute to overindulging in food.
- Eat your meals sitting at a table, away from distractions, if possible.
- Make it a point to have more meals with your spouse or family.

- Develop the habit of eating just when you're really hungry and stopping when you're pleasantly full.
- Reduce your portion sizes by 20% or give up second helpings entirely to lose weight.
- Make use of low-fat dairy products.
- Replace mayonnaise with mustard and whole-grain bread to make sandwiches that are more filling and nutritious.
- Make a cafe au lait instead of a latte by using strong coffee and heated skim milk instead of cream.
- A healthy lunch or snack every few hours should be included in your daily routine.
- Cooking using nonstick cookware and cooking spray instead of oil may help you lose weight while eating healthier.
- Experiment with a variety of cooking techniques, including grilling, roasting, baking, and poaching.
- Increase your water consumption and reduce your intake of sugary beverages.
- Increase your water intake by consuming fewer quantities of calorie-dense items (such as casseroles and pizza) and bigger portions of water-dense foods (like broth-based soups, salads, and veggies).
- Instead of using fatty sauces, use herbs, vinegars, mustards, or lemon to flavour your dish instead.
- Limit your intake of alcoholic beverages to 1-2 drinks each day.

5.2.2 Develop a more mindful attitude

Making a conscious effort to pay more attention to what you eat and drink is one of the first steps in overcoming unhealthy eating habits. Read food labels, get acquainted with ingredient lists, and begin to pay attention to everything you put into your mouth, advises Dr. Gans. Once you become more conscious of what you're eating, you'll be able to see how you can make improvements to your eating habits. Some individuals find it beneficial to maintain meal diaries.

5.2.3 Make a plan and be specific about it

How are you planning to start eating more fruits, having breakfast every day, or going to the gym on a more consistent basis? Make a list of your possibilities. As an illustration: Take an apple to work every day for a snack, stock up on cereal and fruit for quick breakfasts, and visit the gym on your way to work three times a week. "Saying things like 'I'm going to work out more' will not assist you," says Gans. Thinking about when and how you can fit it into your schedule can be beneficial, says the author.

5.2.4 Set a new mini-goal for yourself every week

Eventually, all of these little movements will add up to a significant shift. Example: If your aim is to eat more veggies, commit to trying one new vegetable each week until you discover one that you truly love eating. Consider finding simple methods to include one more serving of veggies into your diet each week until you accomplish your goal. Adding thinly sliced cucumbers to your lunch sandwich, shredded carrots to your morning muffins, or sun-dried tomatoes and mushrooms to your supper pizza are all good ideas.

5.2.5 be realistic in your expectations

Don't set yourself up for failure by expecting too much too quickly. It takes around one month for any new behaviour to become habitual. Slow and steady wins the race — as well as a healthy dosage of attentiveness — every time.

5.2.6 Develop a stress management strategy

As Foreyt suggests, "concentrate on coping with stress in a healthy way via exercise, relaxation, meditation, or whatever method works best for you, so that you don't fall back into old patterns during times of stress or turn to food to help you cope with the issue."

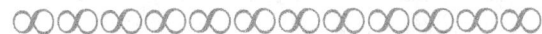

Chapter No. 06

Good Habits that's makes life healthy

6.1   Elements of a well-balanced existence

It is reliant on two components to maintain a healthy equilibrium, which are as follows:

- Consume a nutritious and well-balanced diet.
- Exercises to Help You Maintain Your Balance

6.2   The importance of a healthy diet in living a healthy lifestyle

An effective diet that is well-balanced cannot be overstated when it comes to keeping a healthy lifestyle. Following a well-balanced diet and keeping in mind the importance of providing the body with all of the essential nutrients it need to operate correctly will help you live a healthier lifestyle. Maintaining a healthy body weight and lowering the chance of developing chronic diseases like diabetes, cardiovascular disease, and numerous types of cancer are both made easier with a well-designed meal plan.

What precisely is a well-balanced diet, and how does one achieve one?

In particular, what is a "balanced diet," and how does one go about achieving one? In layman's words, it is a diet that supplies your body with the nutrients it needs to function properly and efficiently. An essential aspect of diet is that it guarantees that the proper amount of calories is eaten. The nutrients your body needs to operate effectively are provided by foods that are rich in calories, such as fresh fruits and vegetables, whole grains, and lean meats.

6.2.1 Calories

Calories are a unit of measurement for the amount of energy contained in a certain quantity of food. Once you've had the meal, the calories are wasted in a variety of ways, such as when you move, think, or breathe. In order to maintain their present body weight on average, a person may need around 2000 calories per day. A person's caloric intake may be modified by their gender, age, and amount of physical activity, among other factors. In addition, males have a larger caloric need than females. For the second time, those who participate in higher physical activity need more calories than those who do not. It's vital to remember that the source of calories is equally as significant as the total quantity of calories you take in one day. Filling your diet with empty calories, that is, calories that have no nutritional value, will have no effect on your weight loss efforts. Empty calories may be found in a wide range of foods, including the following:

- Sugar
- Butter
- Cookies
- Cakes
- Drinks that have a lot of energy
- Ice cream is a delicious treat.
- Pizza

6.3 The importance of eating a well-balanced diet,

In order to feel good and have more energy, as well as to enhance your health and the overall quality of your life, eating a nutritious diet is the objective. Regular physical activity and the maintenance of a healthy body weight are all critical components of a person's overall health and well-being.

In order to live a healthy life, it is unquestionably necessary to consume nutritious meals. The importance of a nutritious food for a healthy body cannot be overstated, since it makes you less prone to illnesses, infections, and even fatigue. Because children are more prone to a range of growth and developmental challenges if they do not eat enough nutritious food, it is especially vital to highlight the need of consuming enough nutritious food for children. Heart disease, cancer, stroke, and diabetes are just a few of the health problems that may arise as a consequence of eating a bad diet that is not properly balanced in its nutrients.

Stress, sadness, and pain levels are reduced as a result of physical exercise, which helps to manage a broad variety of health disorders as well as boost mental wellness. A regular exercise plan may aid in the prevention of metabolic syndrome as well as heart disease, high blood pressure, arthritis, and anxiety problems, among other things.

3.4 What precisely falls within the heading of a well-balanced diet

In order to be considered a "balanced diet," certain specific healthy food categories must be included in the diet. These food categories are as follows: The vegetables leafy greens, starchy vegetables, legumes such as beans and peas, red and orange vegetables, and other vegetables such as eggplant are examples of foods that are considered vegetables.

Fruits that are composed of whole fruits, fresh or frozen fruits, but not canned fruits that have been soaked in syrup, are permitted. Complex carbohydrates are found in grains such as whole grains and refined grains, among other things. Granules that are rich in protein include, for example, quinoa; oats; brown rice; barley; and buckwheat; among other grains. Protein-rich foods include lean meats and poultry, as well as fowl, fish, beans, peas, and legumes, among other things. Calcium may be found in dairy products such as low-fat milk, yoghurt, cottage cheese, and soy milk, among other things.

The nutritional alternatives given should include a diverse selection from each of the five food groups in the proportions recommended by the American Dietetic Association (ADA). They are a good source of energy since they provide a similar number of key micro and macronutrients to meet the body's requirements for these nutrients, despite the fact that they come from different dietary categories. According to experts, a well-balanced diet has 50 to 60 percent carbohydrates, 12 to 20 percent protein, and 30 percent fat. In order for the organs and tissues to operate effectively, they need appropriate nutrition. This is accomplished by consuming the necessary amount of nutrients and calories to maintain a healthy weight and body composition. The importance of a person's general health and well-being may be attributed to many aspects, including food, physical exercise, and maintaining a healthy body weight.

For each age group, a good meal pattern consists of a well-balanced combination of the nutritional components, food items, and serving sizes that are required for each of the four meals. To grow muscle mass, all that is required is protein, as well as blood cells to carry oxygen and nutrients to and from your muscles. In order to maintain physical health and well-being, the body need high-quality carbohydrates, lean protein, essential fats, and water, all of which must be accompanied with regular physical activity.

Healthier lives, on the other hand, are associated with improved sleep and happiness, as well as the avoidance of excessive weight gain or the maintenance of weight loss achieved via exercise. Physical activity, in particular, has been proven to improve brain-related function and outcomes in a variety of studies. It is possible that little changes to your diet, similar to those you would make to your physical activity, may make a major impact in your ability to attain your ideal body weight. It is critical to eat the correct kind of carbohydrates for your needs. Simple carbs, such as those found in sugary snacks and processed foods, are essential for many individuals.

Produce such as fruits and vegetables is a rich source of natural fiber, vitamins, minerals, and other nutrients that your body need in order to function properly and maintain good health. Aside from that, they are very low in calories and fat. The consumption of unsaturated fats, while supplying calories, may be advantageous in lowering inflammation in the body.

6.5 The relevance of keeping a healthy way of living

It is not only required to consume a well-balanced diet, but it is also vital to practice good eating habits in order to achieve this. You may want to consider following some of the following:

- Eat in smaller amounts - you may do this by splitting your meal into little servings, which can trick your brain into thinking you are eating larger portions.
- If you're eating in between other chores, consider eating slowly so that your meals are well-balanced and healthy and your brain recognizes that you've consumed enough calories to keep you going.
- Cut down on unhealthy snacks, which should be avoided at all costs since they have a negative impact on appetite. Making the adjustment to bite-sized meals that are high in nutrition may be advantageous.
- Reduce emotional eating - Binge eating has been shown to be very detrimental to one's general health. Use of marijuana to relieve stress, grief, or concern may have a harmful influence on your health, so use with caution. As an alternative, you may use more healthy coping mechanisms to cope with your unwanted sensations.

3.6   Eating habits are beneficial to your overall health

In order to enhance your general well-being, it is necessary to include healthy eating habits into your daily routine. However, although trendy diets and lifestyle overhauls are now all the rage, the fact is that little modifications and replacements may have a huge influence on one's overall health and well-being.

Because I am a licensed dietitian, my go-to healthy-eating recommendations are those that I provide to people who want to consume more nutritious foods. Almost all of my recommendations are simple to put into action, and they do not need the use of expensive supplements or juice cleanses in order to be effective. Generally speaking, I recommend that people choose two or three healthy eating habit adjustments to kick-start their healthy eating journey, in order to make the changes more durable and long-lasting. Once you've mastered a few methods, you may begin to broaden your skill set and increase your repertory.

Here are the top 20 healthy eating habits that have been approved by dietitians and have been found to have a substantial impact on one's overall health for people who are serious about making positive changes in their eating habits.

6.6.1 Stay away from drinks that include added sugars

Many beverages that seem to be healthy, such as fruit punch and sports drinks, in fact contain hidden sugars that are not readily apparent. Obesity, cardiovascular disease, type 2 diabetes, nonalcoholic fatty liver disease, and metabolic syndrome are just a few of the harmful consequences of eating an excessive quantity of added sugar, according to research. Dietary Guidelines for Americans recommend that people limit their added sugar intake to less than 10% of their total calorie intake. It would take around 12 tablespoons of the sweet stuff to meet a 2,000-calorie diet, according to the nutrition facts. Despite this, the average daily intake of added sugars among persons in the United States is around 17 teaspoons, which is far more than the recommended maximum. Drinking sugary beverages (such as conventional soda and sweet tea) in moderation and substituting sugar-free alternatives (such as water, seltzer water, unsweetened coffee or tea) can help you get the hydration your body needs to function properly.

6.6.2 Include fermented foods in your diet

Live probiotics found in fermented foods such as kimchee, sauerkraut, and other fermented foods not only taste good, but they also feed the body with helpful bacteria that are useful to our overall health in a variety of ways. Drink kombucha in the middle of the day or have plain yoghurt for breakfast to give your body a boost of probiotics and other healthy microorganisms.

6.6.3 Reduce your mercury intake by eating

Despite the fact that the Dietary Guidelines for Americans indicate that most Americans eat at least 8 ounces of fish each week, the overwhelming majority of people do not consume the required quantity. Foods containing omega-3 fatty acids, especially oily fish such as salmon, are a wonderful source of DHA omega-3 fatty acids as well as other essential nutrients that are helpful to human health, including selenium, vitamin B12, and a multitude of other trace elements. People who eat fish seem to live an average of 2.2 years longer than those who do not consume fish, according to the research. As an added bonus, eating fish has been linked to a decreased chance of developing type 2 diabetes as well as heart disease (CVD).

6.6.4 Reduce the amount of processed meat

Highly processed meats such as lunch meats, bacon, and sausage are unquestionably convenient, but they are also very appetizing to consume in large quantities. These meat alternatives, on the other hand, may be rich in nitrates, a component that, when cooked, may produce compounds that are possibly harmful to people. On top of all that, a lot of these meat selections are also heavy in salt, which is not a good thing. It is feasible to consume fresh cuts of meat such as turkey, chicken, and beef that are lower in sodium and nitrates while still being delicious to eat and enjoy.

6.6.5 Consume at least one glass of milk daily

Milk isn't only for newborns and toddlers any more, though. It contains 13 essential nutrients, including calcium, protein, and magnesium, all of which are important to bone health. A glass of milk is a simple meal that makes a fantastic partner to chocolate chip cookies. Despite the fact that milk is very healthy, only around 20% of the population consumes even a single glass of this beverage each day, according to the Centers for Disease Control and Prevention.

6.6.6 Incorporate fruits and vegetables

Only one out of every ten Americans eats the recommended daily amounts of fruits and vegetables, according to the USDA. More importantly, since decreasing fruit consumption is related with unfavourable repercussions such as an increased risk for some cancers, heart disease, and stroke, sneaking in a piece of fruit every day is a sensible choice. In order to avoid reaching for sugary snacks or caffeine-laden beverages when the afternoon slump hits, make fruit part of your balanced snack. Fruit may provide you with prolonged energy as well as nutrients that help you stay energized throughout the rest of the day, so include it in your balanced snack. You may assist guarantee that your snack has lasting power and that you will feel satisfied rather than having a sugar crash shortly after eating by pairing one or two servings of fruit with one or two servings of protein.

Keep in mind that if you don't have access to fresh fruit, dried, freeze-dried, and frozen fruit are all healthful alternatives, as long as they don't have any added salt or sugar (or both). As a consequence, dried fruits are now accessible in a wide array of varieties, ranging from freeze-dried blueberries to dried mango slices.

6.6.7 Increase the amount of veggies in meal.

Fiber-rich veggies are a fantastic source of nutrition for your body, as they may assist to keep your body healthy by maintaining intestinal health and perhaps decreasing your chance of acquiring some malignancies. Foods such as vegetables are also one of the most abundant sources of vitamin C, which may assist to keep your body healthy by lowering your chances of acquiring some malignancies. Furthermore, many veggies are low in calories and may be utilized to make recipes a bit more substantial and tasty by substituting them for other vegetables in the dish.

Aside from the fact that you should include vegetables in your recipes, you should not eat salad for every meal of the day. A handful of spinach or additional broccoli may be added to your stir-fry or a cup of soup for a fast and simple method to give your food a healthy boost.

6.6.8 Prevent eating in front of the television

It is meant to allow you to have pleasure in your meals. Furthermore, when you eat while watching television, you may become distracted, which may result in you consuming more calories. This is because research has shown that watching television can interfere with various processes that are typically involved in the voluntary management of food intake, such as appetite suppression and food intake control. In lieu of this, get together with friends and family to enjoy your meals together. Alternatively, ensure that you are not distracted by the television while you are eating. Alternatively,

6.6.9 Choose canned foods

Because they are readily available and simple to prepare, healthy canned foods such as tuna and beans are simple to include into a well-balanced diet. However, if the cans in which your food is stored contain BPA, a chemical that assists in the prevention of metal corrosion, it is possible that you are not eating as healthfully as you think.

Despite the fact that the FDA maintains there is insufficient evidence that BPA from cans is harmful, some studies have linked higher BPA levels to an increased risk of type 2 diabetes, obesity, high blood pressure, and other unfavorable outcomes, according to the FDA. The majority of automobile manufacturers in the United States have voluntarily halted the use of bisphenol A (BPA), but there is concern that similar replacement compounds may also be harmful to human health. At this time, the quantity of known research on the safety of these options is inadequate to make a conclusive decision. Last but not least, if you're concerned about the environmental impact of these materials, go for things that are packed in glass or aseptic paper containers.

6.6.10 Make a plan for your daily meals

Individuals who plan their meals are more likely to consume a nutritious diet and, if they are overweight, are more likely to lose weight as well. Spending the time and effort to plan your meals for the week will make it much more difficult to adhere to a healthy eating plan during the week. To meal plan, you must first decide what you will eat for each of your seven daily meals throughout the week before you can begin. By creating a shopping list and putting together the ingredients for fast dinners for the full week ahead of time, you may save time and money.

6.6.11 Prevent yourself from eating the same things

Having the capacity to eat a variety of foods is critical for keeping a healthy lifestyle. Dietary diversity will offer your body with a variety of nutrients and may aid in the prevention of nutritional deficiency. As a result of these findings, it has been hypothesized that eating a varied variety of healthful meals may reduce the chance of developing metabolic syndrome. Eat foods that naturally include a range of colors throughout the week, according to an approach advised by many dietitians and known as "eating the rainbow," according to many dietitians. Each kind of coloured vegetable, such as purple cabbage and carrots, scarlet radish or spinach, is helpful to one's health in its own way; nevertheless, the nutritional composition of each variety differs. Changing around the foods on your plate may keep things interesting while also ensuring that your body receives a range of critical nutrients on a continuous basis.

6.6.12 preparing your veggies

It is best to prepare your veggies before keeping them in the refrigerator before putting your groceries away after your shopping excursion. Incorporating fresh vegetables into your cooking, such as finely chopped onions and thinly sliced cucumbers, makes it easier to include healthful vegetables into your diet.

6.6.13 Avoid drinking diet soda

With no calories and a naturally sweet taste, it makes logical sense to suppose that ingesting diet Coke is an excellent choice for weight loss. In fact, according to recent study, drinking diet Coke may really be more harmful to your health than you previously thought. The bubbly, sugary beverage may actually increase your risk of developing cardiovascular disease. According to the results of a second study, people with type 2 diabetes who drink more than four cans of diet soda each week are more likely to develop vision difficulties.

6.6.14 Limit your intake of fried meals to a minimum

There is nothing quite like the experience of biting into a crispy French fry or a piece of crispy fried chicken. Consuming an excessive quantity of fried meals, on the other hand, has been associated to a number of undesirable health consequences.

To create that wonderful crunch without the extra calories and fat of deep-frying or baking, try air-frying or baking your foods instead of deep-frying or baking.

6.6.16 In place of beverages, mock tails may be used

Consumption of alcoholic drinks may increase the risk of acquiring some types of cancer, including prostate cancer. Some individuals, on the other hand, may find that giving up their nightly drink represents a substantial shift in their life. Many individuals like the ritual of sipping on a pleasant beverage, and mock tails are an excellent method to decrease or eliminate alcohol intake while still participating in the ritual of sipping on a tasty beverage.

6.6.16 save money, use thinner cuts of meat

In addition to being a naturally occurring source of iron, protein, zinc, and a range of other necessary nutrients, beef may be included in a nutritious diet. Moreover, although some cuts of beef are higher in saturated fat than others, leaner cuts, such as flank steak, are perfectly fine as part of a nutritious diet when consumed in moderation as part of a well-balanced diet.

6.6.17 Utilize beans

If you follow a balanced diet, beans may be one of the most nutritious foods you may include in it, regardless of whether you are a carnivore or a committed vegan. There are a variety of factors contributing to this. The fact that they are a plant-based, cost-effective source of protein that is both versatile and enjoyable to consume speaks volumes about their nutritional value. Beans have a combination of total and soluble fiber as well as resistant starch, both of which contribute to their low glycemic index and low calorie content. Furthermore, they contain polyphenols, many of which are effective antioxidants, making them a healthy choice. If you consume beans on a regular basis as part of a well-balanced diet, you may be able to lower your LDL ("bad") cholesterol levels and reduce your risk of developing diabetes.

6.6.18 don't forget to eat your breakfast

Everybody knows that breakfast is regarded to be the most important meal of the day, and we all agree that this is true. Moreover, a recent research has shown exactly why this is the case. In this study, eating breakfast on a consistent basis was shown to be connected with a greater intake of a range of nutrients such as folate, calcium, iron, and zinc. The data also found that those who skip breakfast consume much more calories, carbohydrates, total and saturated fat, and added sugars during the rest of the day than people who have a nutritious breakfast every day.

6.6.19 Avoid depriving yourself of the foods

Even if you are attempting to live a healthy lifestyle, it is not recommended that you consume a dozen doughnuts or one gallon of ice cream on a daily basis. On the other hand, if you deprive yourself of your favourite meals all at once, you can find yourself overindulging in the long run. Every now and then, you should treat yourself to something delicious to help you keep satisfied and on track with your weight reduction objectives. Treating yourself to a treat now and then is OK as long as you are consuming a decent amount of the food and doing it in moderation.

3.6.20 Feasible, use herbs

American adults eat an average of around 3,400 milligrams of salt per day, despite the fact that the Dietary Guidelines recommend no more than 2,300 milligrams of sodium per day for adults. Increased risk of developing hypertension is associated with excessive salt consumption on a regular basis. Reduce your sodium consumption by limiting the quantity of salt you use in your meals, according to the American Heart Association. One teaspoon of table salt contains more than 2,000 milligrams of sodium, making it a good spot to begin your sodium reduction journey. It is recommended that you use flavorful additions such as herbs and spices that are sodium-free yet still pack a flavor punch while attempting to lower your salt intake.

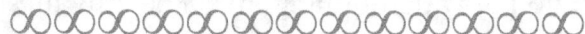

Chapter No. 07

Lose Weight without Going on a Diet

In fact, losing weight in a short period of time is possible. The internet is full of fad diets that promise to help you lose weight quickly while also leaving you feeling hungry and depleted. If you are just going to get it back, then what is the point of reducing weight in the first place? Weight loss should be done gradually in order to maintain weight loss over the long term... The vast majority of professionals believe that this is doable without resorting to "diet" methods. As an alternative, it is vital to make little adjustments to your way of life to achieve success.

A pound of fat has around 3,500 calories. A pound of fat has around 3,500 calories. A weekly weight reduction of around one pound may be achieved by increasing your calorie intake by 500 calories per day by dietary and activity adjustments, respectively. The simple act of cutting 100 calories from your daily calorie intake will assist you avoid gaining the 1-2 pounds that the majority of individuals acquire each year. Simply reducing your daily calorie consumption by 100 calories would be sufficient if all you wanted to do was maintain your present weight. Using easy, painless techniques of reducing weight without having to go on a "diet" may be beneficial for people of all ages and physical fitness levels.

- Eat breakfast at least once a day, preferably twice. Many people who have been successful in losing weight and keeping it off have acquired the habit of eating breakfast every morning. Author Elizabeth Ward, MS, RD, who co-authored The Pocket Idiot's Guide to the New Food Pyramids, says that although many individuals believe that skipping breakfast is a great way to lose weight, they actually end up consuming more calories throughout the day as a consequence of their choice. The author of the study said that "many folks believe that skipping breakfast is a terrific method to reduce calories," but that "they typically wind up eating more during the day." People who eat breakfast have lower BMIs than those who do not, and they do better in school and in the boardroom, according to research findings. Additionally, they have reduced cholesterol levels. A bowl of whole-grain cereal topped with fruit and low-fat dairy products is a fast and healthy dinner option for those on the go.
- Keep the kitchen door closed at all times over the course of the evening. Avoiding late-night cravings or mindless munching in front of the television by scheduling a time when you will be done eating is

essential. Having a cup of tea after dinner, sucking on a hard candy, or consuming a small bowl of light ice cream or frozen yoghurt as an after-dinner treat are all suggestions made by Elaine Magee, the "Recipe Doctor" and author of Comfort Food Makeovers. "Having a cup of tea with a piece of hard candy or having a small dish of light ice cream after supper are all good options if you're looking for something sweet. "However, she adds, "brushing your teeth first will make you less likely to ingest more meals and liquids," according to her."

- Select Liquid Calories as the calorie type from the drop-down menu that appears. Wisely. Despite the fact that sweetened beverages are heavy in calories, they do not deliver the same amount of hunger satisfaction as substantial meals. You may quench your thirst by consuming simple water, sparkling water with citrus, skim or low-fat milk, or little quantities of 100 percent fruit juice to meet your requirements. If you find yourself becoming hungry in between meals or as a snack, try a glass of nutritious and low-calorie vegetable juice to keep you going. Make sure to keep an eye on your alcohol calories, since they may rapidly build up if you drink too much of it. If you like a glass or two of wine or a cocktail on most days, restricting your alcohol use to the weekends will help you lose weight and lose weight quickly, which is particularly beneficial if you are overweight.

- Consume a greater range of fruits and vegetables to increase your consumption of these nutrients. 5. Because of their large volume and low calorie content, increased consumption of low-calorie, high-volume fruits and vegetables may aid in reducing consumption of other foods that are higher in fat and calories as a consequence of their low calorie content and high volume. Remove the meat from the middle of your plate and put a mountain of veggies on top of it to make a mountain of vegetables. According to Barbara Rolls, PhD, the inventor of The Volumetric Eating Plan, a vegetable salad or a bowl of broth-based soup may be provided before lunch or dinner instead of a meal. Americans should consume 7-13 cups of fresh vegetables per day, according to the Dietary Guidelines for Americans, published in 2005. "Stuff your kitchen with a variety of fruits and veggies, and include a few of these products into every meal and snack," Ward suggests if you want to achieve this goal. You will benefit from include more super-nutritious vegetables and less processed foods in your diet since your diet will be richer in vitamins, minerals, phytonutrients, and fiber as a result, and you will be less likely to go for the cookie jar as a result of doing so.

- Make judgments based on the grain of information available to you. Whole grains may be substituted for refined grains such as white bread, cakes, pastries, and pretzels to boost the amount of fiber in your diet while also filling you full more quickly, making it easier to consume a healthy number of calories per day. When it comes to carbs, whole-wheat bread and pasta (or brown rice), bran flakes (or popcorn), and whole-rye crackers are all good options to consider (or a combination of the above).
- Maintain your ability to exercise control over your environment. It is also possible to control your surroundings, which may include anything from filling your kitchen with plenty of healthy alternatives to picking the correct eateries, to aid you in reducing weight. As part of this, stay away from buffets and other similar establishments to avoid being tempted and overindulging in unhealthy foods. For further advice, Ward recommends that you "have a nutritious snack before a party so that you won't be hungry, and exercise prudence while heaping your plate at the buffet," according to Ward. Make sure to wait 15 minutes and drink a large glass of water before returning for additional meals.
- Reduce the portion size of the servings that are served. Reduce your portion sizes by 10% to 20% and you will be able to lose weight without

changing your diet or doing anything else. Food provided in restaurants and at home is often far larger than what is required to feed oneself on a regular basis. Measure your typical portion sizes using the measuring cups in order to have a better knowledge of them and to begin working on reducing them as soon as possible. According to Dr. Brian Wansink (author of the book Mindless Eating), utilizing tiny bowls, plates, and cups may assist you in developing better portion control more rapidly than using larger serving dishes. Due to the fact that the meal will seem to be plenty on excellent serving dishes, it is doubtful that you would be hungry.

- Include any other measures that you plan to take. Make the purchase of a pedometer and progressively raise the number of steps you walk each day until you reach a daily total of 10,000 or more steps each day During the course of the day, make every attempt to be more physically active - take a stroll around the house while you're on the phone, take the dog for an extra walk, or march in place during commercial breaks on television. Using a pedometer on a regular basis provides an ongoing motivation and acts as a reminder to engage in increased physical activity.

- Make sure that protein is included in each and every meal and snack you consume. Incorporating a portion of lean or low-fat protein into each meal and snack can help you feel satisfied for longer periods of time, which may lower your chances of overindulging during those meals and snacks. Low-fat yoghurt, a little quantity of nuts or peanut butter, and eggs, lentils, and lean meats are all wonderful options for a healthy breakfast. Experts suggest eating small but frequent meals and snacks (every 3-4 hours) to keep blood glucose levels steady and to prevent overindulging in sugary or high-carbohydrate foods, according to the American Diabetes Association.

- Make the switch to more environmentally friendly replacements for your items as soon as possible. The quantity of fat you consume on a daily basis may be reduced by picking low-fat salad dressings, mayonnaise, dairy products, and other items from the grocery store. It is possible to simply cut your calorie consumption by consuming low-fat and lighter foods, and if the product is blended in with other components, no one will be the wiser, according to Magee. Consuming low-fat and lighter foods, says Magee, can help you to cut your calorie consumption quickly and effortlessly. Here are a few additional suggestions for imaginative substitutes to think about: Rather of sprinkling on the creamy dressing, reduce the amount of cheese on your sandwiches and pour a little vinaigrette over your salad, rather than spreading it on.

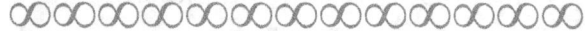

Chapter No. 08

Exercises that make you Healthy

8.1   Push-ups

Please drop and give me a twenty-dollar bill! For those looking for body-weight workouts that are both simple and effective, pushups are a great choice. They activate a huge variety of muscles, making it one of the most basic and effective exercises available. To begin, take a plank position on the ground. In order to maintain a neutral posture, your abdominal muscles should be tight and your shoulders should be brought down and back.

Starting from the floor, bend your elbows and slowly lower your body to the surface of the floor. Return to the starting position as soon as your chest makes contact with the bar. Throughout the workout, keep your elbows close to your body and your wrists as relaxed as possible. Complete three sets of as many repetitions as you are able in a certain time frame. To accomplish a normal pushup with good form, establish a modified stance on your knees and push yourself up. You will still enjoy the most of the advantages of this workout while also strengthening your overall physical strength.

4.2   Squats

When you lift your legs up and down, you build lower-body strength and core stability while also developing flexibility in your low-back and hip joints. Because they include the activation of some of the largest muscles in the body, they also result in a considerable increase in calorie expenditure as a result of their involvement. Maintain a straight stance, with your feet slightly wider than shoulder width apart and your arms relaxed at your sides, as seen in the photo. In the same way you would if you were going to sit down in a chair, brace your core and maintain proper posture by keeping your chest and chin up while pushing your hips back and knees bent. Extend your arms out in front of you in a comfortable stance, then lower yourself until your thighs are parallel to the ground, maintaining your knees from bowing inward or outward. After one second of pause, return to the starting position and extend your legs before repeating the procedure.

Completing three sets of 20 repetitions is recommended.

8.3   Dumbbell

Compound exercises, which involve the use of multiple joints and muscles, are ideal for people who lead busy lives because they train multiple sections of the body at the same time. Compound exercises are particularly beneficial for people who lead busy lives because they train multiple sections of the body at the same time. A standing overhead press is not just one of the most effective shoulder exercises you can do, but it also strengthens your upper back and core muscles, which are all important for overall health.

It is necessary to use dumbbells that weigh 10 pounds.

For this exercise, we recommend using a low-weight set of dumbbells (we recommend 10 pounds for beginners). Start by standing with your feet shoulder-width apart or staggered, depending on your personal choice. Keep your upper arms parallel to the ground while you raise the weights in the picture above to avoid injury. Continue to push upward, bracing your core as you do so, until your arms are fully extended above your head. Make sure your head and neck are in a stable posture. Bend your elbows and lower the weight back down until your triceps muscle is parallel to the floor once again in the following seconds.

Completing three sets of 12 repetitions is recommended.

8.4   Dumbbell rows

Dumbbell rows, in addition to making your back look fantastic in that dress, are a complicated exercise that serves to train numerous muscles in your upper body at the same time, including the pectorals and triceps.

Make sure you're squeezing at the very top of the movement with a moderate-weight dumbbell before moving on to the next.

It is necessary to use dumbbells that weigh 10 pounds.

To begin, grip a dumbbell in each hand and lift it to your chest. We recommend that beginners use a weight that is no more than 10 pounds in total. It's necessary to lean forward at the waist in order to stretch your back at a 45-degree angle to the ground. Check to see that you are not arching your back. Your arms should be entirely free to hang straight down. Before you begin, check to see that your neck is in alignment with your back and that your core is engaged. Beginning with your right arm, bend your elbow and bring the weight straight up toward your chest, being sure to keep your lats engaged the whole time, terminating just below your chest. Repeat with your left arm. Repeat the process with your left arm.

Once you've returned to the starting position, repeat the same with your left arm. This is the first of many repetitions. Repeat this for a total of three sets of 10 repetitions in each direction.

8.5   Deadlifts performed with just one leg
This is another another exercise that will put your ability to keep your balance to the test once again.

Single-leg deadlifts need stability and leg strength on the lifting leg in order to be effective. You will want a light to moderate dumbbell in order to do this manoeuvre.

To begin, hold a dumbbell in your right hand and slowly bend both legs at the hips to form a V-shape with your legs. Kick your left leg straight back behind you, lowering the dumbbell down toward the ground while hunching at the hips to begin the exercise. In a calm and gentle way, return to the starting position with your left leg after reaching a comfortable height with it. Squeezing the Glute of your right hip will help you do this. As you do the movement, make sure that your pelvis stays square to the ground throughout. Then, moving the weight to your left hand and doing the same steps on your left leg as you did for the right, repeat the process for 10 to 12 repetitions.

8.6   Burpees

Exercises such as burpees are a very effective whole-body exercise that provides you with a great deal of bang for your buck in terms of both aerobic endurance and muscular strength. Despite the fact that we dislike them, they are quite effective. Starting by standing tall with your feet shoulder width apart and your arms down at your sides is a wonderful location to get started with yoga. From a standing position with your hands out in front of you, stoop as low as you possibly can. When your hands contact the ground, it's a good idea to straighten your legs and get into a pushup position as quickly as possible.

Jumping your feet up to your palms is made possible by a waistband that is attached at the waist. Reposition your feet as close as possible to your hands, landing them outside of your hands if necessary, and repeat the procedure. With your arms outstretched over your head, leap off the ground and into the air. Maintain a straight posture. This is the first of many repetitions. As a beginner, do three sets of 10 repetitions each.

8.7   Side planks are used

It is critical to maintain a strong core as the structural foundation of your body; consequently, core-specific workouts such as the side plank should not be overlooked. In order to guarantee that you are properly completing this movement, you must concentrate on the connection between your thoughts and your muscles, as well as on creating regulated motions. Lie down with your back straight and your right leg and foot stacked on top of your left leg and foot in a "right-side-up" posture. You may elevate your upper body by resting your right forearm on the ground and your right elbow just under your shoulder on the right side of the body. Because of the core contraction, your spine will be straightened, as will be your hips and knees, which will form a straight line with your body as a consequence of your core contraction. Returning to the beginning of the story on purpose. On one side, do three sets of 10–15 repetitions, then switch to the other side and continue the procedure.

8.8   Planks

In addition to working your core muscles, planks are an excellent technique to engage your complete body at the same time. Planking is a great way to build your core without placing too much tension on your back, like setups and crunches may. As you begin in a pushup posture, make sure your hands and toes are firmly planted on the ground, your back is straight, and your core is taut. Make sure your chin is slightly tucked in, and that your gaze is just in front of the palms of your hands. Keep your tension in your stomach, shoulders, triceps, gluts, and quadriceps by taking deep, controlled breaths and maintaining tension throughout your whole body.

To get started, complete 2-3 sets of 30 second holds to warm up your muscles.

8.9   The bridge of the gluteus

The Glute Bridge is a fantastic exercise because it works your entire posterior chain, which is not only beneficial to your health but also makes your booty appear perkier as a result of the increased activity. A good place to start is by laying down on the floor with your knees bent and your feet flat on the ground, your arms straight at your sides and your palms facing down.

Lift your hips off the ground to complete the movement by pressing through your heels and squeezing your core, gluts, and hamstring muscles. The ground should still be in contact with your upper back and shoulders while you are in this position, and a straight line should be drawn from the middle of your back to your knees during this position. Take a 1–2 second break at the top of the hill, and then return to the starting position.

Complete three sets of ten to twelve repetitions each.

8.10 Pilates

Pilates is a terrific activity that is suitable for beginners and may help you reduce weight.

Following the findings of research sponsored by the American Council on Exercise, an individual weighing around 140 pounds (64 kg) would burn 108 calories during a 30-minute beginner's Pilates session, and 168 calories during an expert Pilate's class of the same length of time. The fact that many individuals find Pilates pleasurable makes it easier to persist with it over time, even if it does not burn as many calories as cardio workouts such as jogging or cycling do.

Research conducted on 37 middle-aged women over eight weeks discovered that completing Pilates movements for 90 minutes three times per week substantially lowered waist, stomach, and hip circumferences when compared to a control group that performed no exercise during the same period. Pilates, in addition to helping you lose weight, has been proved to relieve lower back discomfort while simultaneously improving your strength, balance, flexibility, endurance, and general fitness. If you're interested in giving Pilates a try, consider adding it to your weekly schedule. Pilates may be practiced at home or at one of the numerous gyms that provide Pilates lessons regularly. Combine Pilates with a balanced diet and other types of exercise, such as weight training or cardio, to increase the effectiveness of your weight reduction efforts.

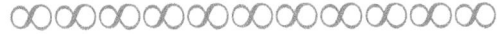